THE FAT-CHANCE DIET

By

Dr. Hans Spud

ISBN: 0-75962-650-2

This book is printed on acid free paper.

1stBooks - rev. 5/8/01

Everywhere one turns these days, there are diets! Dozens upon dozens of books have come out prescribing this or that diet: "The Ragsdale, Illinois Diet" or "The Amazing Yogurt & French Toast Diet." Frankly people are sick of it! (The diets, not the yogurt and French toast, necessarily.)

People are told to eat more of this and less of that, etc. The hefty people of this country are, pardon the expression, fed up. People are ready to call a halt, to stop it short, and to nip it in the bud. The time has come for one final, exhaustive, comprehensive, authoritative diet book to put an end to the balderdash, nonsense, silliness, and poppycock. At long last, in plain English, or something close to it, the truth about diets!

To settle this diet madness once and for all, one of the world's most knowledgeable authorities on human nutrition and the effect of crepes on the human body speak out to set the record straight. Dr. Hans Spud reveals the plain unvarnished trust. Dr. Spud explains in this volume who is fat, what fat is (and is not), how to get incredibly skinny, how to stay fat but appear skinny, how to stay skinny but appear to be fat, and, space permitting, how to samba.

1

Numerous other chapters were prepared for this book, but due to limited space, were deleted. Some of these chapters were really something! Too bad you missed them! You would have learned how to prepare a low-calorie grape quiche, where to find extra-heavy-duty bathroom scales, and how to play rugby. You would have learned how to make a cranberry fondue, speak Portuguese, and mud wrestle, just to mention a very few topics.

If you are among the millions of Americans (or for that matter, some kind of European or Asian) who faces the sad fact that he or she is overweight, fat, heavy, chunky, obese, or portly, and who wants to be thin, sleek, angular, or emaciated, you may find the answers with Dr. Spud. Then again, you may not. But give it a chance. Read the book carefully. Perhaps you will be so busy reading you will forget to eat! All the better! Or, as some do, you may choose to read from the back to the front, which will make you think you are already thin.

AN INTRODUCTION TO FAT AND CHANCE

As a beginning to this subject of the diet, one must forget everything he has learned. At least about diets. This will be much easier if one has learned nothing. We will begin by understanding something of the origin of diet, whirl through a brief but uninformative history of the diet, then back up and attempt to correct whatever we said. Please follow carefully, or you will probably get the instructions all wrong and proceed to grow increasingly fat. I mean FAT. Not just fooling around.

Now, I look at this word "diet." Do you see it? It is believed by some that the word is derived from the Latin "diaeta." If you believe that, you will believe anything!

The earliest reference, indeed, occurred when a Hun cast an enemy into a darkened hole, leaving him there for several weeks, and leaving a guard to watch over him. Not actually, literally, to watch over him. That would have been foolish, wouldn't it? No, rather, the guard watched him, not over him. But let us not be picky. If we are going to quibble over every little thing, we will never get through this book. The point is that the Hun returned daily, peered into the hole, and inquired of the guard, "Die yet?" Through the years the expression was somehow contracted to "diet." Even today, dieters frequently think of themselves as having been thrown in a dark hole to starve to death.

Since that day there apparently have been fat people, and, thus, there have been diets. New World explorers, pirates, adventurers...wherever you turn in history, there have been fat folk. The Aztecs and Incas, of course, were fat. Mercy, were they large! One hardly ever reads about them, though, because the Aztec and Inca writers were fat themselves, and preferred to make no mention of it. See if you can find any.

The early colonists, European royalty, King George, John Smith, Ethan Allen...you guessed it! Most of these people of bygone days are seen to be thin in the portraits that one observes in art galleries and museums. Who would have paid anyone to paint a portrait in which they were portrayed as fat? The more they paid, the thinner they are in the portraits! Some paid so much they can hardly be seen at all.

So much for history! With the coming of the modern day, television, mass distribution of books, etc., has come a rash of diets. And, yes, we find many diets do cause rashes, so watch yourself! Each diet claims to be better than the last. You have seen these so-called diets. Cottage cheese diets! All of the fat people I know eat cottage cheese, and I have concluded that, that is what is making them fat!

When anyone approaches me with a new diet, I will usually do one of three things.

1. Call a policeman.
2. Place a bucket over my head. (This keeps me from hearing them and also cuts down my food consumption. Try it.)
3. Spray him with MACE.

No, the diets you see are not worth the paper they are printed on. Fat, fat people make them up.

After years of study and research, more than I care to remember, (and I don't care to remember many at all), I have settled on the findings of two Chinese doctors, Dr. Lo

Fat and Dr. Charlie Chance, who developed the Fat-Chance Diet. Now, this Fat-Chance Diet is actually a number of dietary approaches, and in this book we (I should have said I, as you are not helping at all) shall look at a number of these diets which make up the Fat-Chance Diet study. Then we will, after all the others are tried, resort to the Amazing 30-Day-Fat-Chance Diet. If we don't get that far, it means of course that either we have lost the weight we wish or we have died. Probably we (or I should say you) will have died. No, we only kid you.

Most of this presentation, as we said, draws on the conclusions made by Fat and Chance. Some draws on my own experimentation, and some draws on nothing at all. You can decide for yourself which is which.

I might add that Dr. Fat and Dr. Chance are slim and svelte. I will not add that, though, because they are both on the heavy side. In fact, not just on the side. However, they do claim to know how to get thin, and say that they could get skinny if they chose to.

Remember, again, as you begin this book, to forget all the foolish diets you have read about up to now. I laugh at them! Fat and Chance laugh at them. (On more than one occasion I have seen Fat and Chance sit around reading diets, laughing until tears ran from their eyes, and rolling about on the floor. Remember, they were rather heavy themselves, and rolled rather easily.)

Fat and Chance developed their system through three methods, primarily:

1. They observed people. Whenever anyone really fat was in the area, they would come running, poking the persons in the abdomen, examining the food in his lunchsack, and generally making nuisances of themselves. Fat and Chance not only discovered a great deal about the diet of fat people, but also that fat people, when relentlessly aggravated, will become violent.

2. Fat and Chance also reached their conclusions through experimentation. They would mix, say, cod liver oil with chocolate milk, or some such concoction, then make each other drink them. Sometimes, if the concoction were just too terrible, too absolutely yucky, to try, one or the other would refuse to drink it, and hide, perhaps under a bed, or

drive away not to be seen for several weeks. Their research took a long time because of that.

3.   Their third method in establishing their theories was merely to make them up.

Now, you know Fat and Chance as well as anyone. So, we have killed so much time with the introduction, you are probably famished. Go get something to eat, then come back and we will begin. (We will begin with the Amazing Running Diet. We begin with it because it is first.)

THE AMAZING RUNNING DIET

This is the most simple diet of all. Here is how it works:

Eat anything you wish! That is correct, eat whatever you like. Can you believe what your eyes see here? But, aha! Whatever is eaten must be eaten while you are running. Now, when we say "run" what do we mean? We mean, of course, moving one foot ahead of the other very rapidly. You already know what it is to walk. Do that same thing, only make your body go faster. You will find this diet works because it is practically impossible to eat at all while running, especially let's say, a bowl of cereal. (For one thing, the spoon will continually bang against your teeth, make a hellacious racket.)

To test this diet, we followed one large man whom we shall call R.P. of Akron, Ohio, who agreed to try the diet. As he left his suburban home last February 16, at precisely 7:29 a.m., heading in a westerly direction down Oak Street, Dr.'s Fat and Chance and I followed in a plain, black unmarked sedan. Immediately upon leaving his doorway, R.P. burst into a run, or at least a lope of sorts, this 384-

pound man carrying a large bag of groceries. He had gone perhaps eight feet when he became hungry, and reached inside the bag for a cluster of grapes, which slipped from his hand, and bounced, individually, in various directions along the avenue. Huffing and puffing, R.P. continued on, and before reaching the first corner, tried for a Danish roll. Now, bathed in perspiration, R.P. somehow let the roll slip from his hand. It commenced to roll along the sidewalk some feet ahead of R.P. Then, perhaps due to a sudden burst of wind, (we will never know, for certain), the roll bounced over the curb and into what I believe was 23rd Street. R.P. followed the roll as fast as his legs could carry him, and, we are sad to report, was struck by an Akron taxicab. At last report, R.P. was still in Akron General Hospital, but doing well.

The point is that R. P. has lost thirty-five pounds.

We said this was the simplest diet; we did <u>not</u> say it was the <u>easiest</u> diet.

There are other dangers with this diet and it is proper that we set these forth for you. As in most diets, it is possible for one to be carried away, and to overdo it, making a complete fool of yourself. Take the case of Mrs.

C.M. of Brooklyn, New York. Again, as a test case, she agreed as R.P. had, to try the Amazing Running Diet. Again, Drs. Fat and Chance and I proceeded to follow her at a respectable distance. (This time in a yellow 1950 Volkswagen. The black sedan was in the shop.)

After jogging several blocks, Mrs. C.M. began enjoying the run so much that she paused long enough to place the bag of groceries on the sidewalk, and proceeded to run on without them. For a large woman, she was remarkably fast! Never have I seen anyone enjoy running so much! We lost her as she went through the Lincoln Tunnel, and so far as we know, she has not been seen since. Her husband, whom we shall call J.M., did tell us that a few days ago, a woman was spotted running along the New Jersey Turnpike, at a rapid, rapid pace. If this, indeed, was Mrs. C.M., we have reason to believe the diet is successful, as the New Jersey Turnpike authorities describe the woman as having been a rather "slim" woman.

THE AMAZING BLINDFOLD DIET

The Amazing Blindfold Diet was developed quite by accident. No one would have thought of it on purpose. How it was developed by Fat and Chance is not especially interesting, but we will tell it anyway. Fat and Chance, it seems, were attending a cocktail party in California. No, it doesn't <u>seem</u> that they were attending a party. They <u>were</u> attending a party.

Well, to make a long story worse, one of the party games was pin-the-tail-on-the-donkey. Fat, who may have had a bit too much punch, placed the blindfold over his eyes, and proceeded to stagger around the room, madly waving a tail, and eventually pinned the tail on Chance.

When the pain subsided, Chance remarked about how impaired one's vision is when wearing a blindfold. He also remarked about the several other things, but we shall not repeat them here. But, as we say, the blindfold idea struck with him, as did the tail for some while.

Later, when they again were speaking to each other, Fat and Chance decided that they could take the dieter, secure a blindfold around the head, and let him loose to eat anything he wished. When wearing a blindfold, they found, one is very cautious and slow about one's eating. Another tactic recommended by the doctor is the wearing of a clothespin on the nose. This eliminates cheating by smelling food. It also eliminates friends, however. When one answers the door (if he can find it) wearing a blindfold and a clothespin on one's nose, one can expect a cool reception, if he is lucky enough to get one at all. Well, what did you expect? A diet on a silver platter? An easy, pleasant little diet? Any diet that promises you that also promises you that you will stay fat.

The Amazing Blindfold Diet works! Time for another case history, if you can stand it. We have a letter from N.D. of Blue Ridge, Tennessee. Well, not from N.D. himself, as he is still blindfolded, and any letter from him would look like henscratching. It is from his wife, whom we shall call Mrs. N.D. But she relates N.D.'s experience, and why should we doubt her? Give us a good reason. N.D. has gone from 265 pounds to 140 in less than six weeks! At first N.D. was rather cocky, his wife writes, and would try to eat to beat the band. He slowed down considerably when he ate up six pair of shoestrings, thinking he was eating spaghetti. If you choose to try this diet, heed N.D.'s advice and do not go about stuffing things into your mouth at random. But, as a safety precaution, you may wish to have the shoestrings removed from all the shoes in the house.

One other word of wisdom. Keep more or less to yourself. Preferably more. Socialize only with friends and immediate family. With the blindfold and clothespin in place, one can easily be taken in by a prankster. One large woman (from Gary, Indiana, file number 76044) spent the better part of an evening trying to cut up a "pot roast" that turned out to be nothing more than an old catcher's mitt.

THE AMAZING HYPNOTISM DIET

You have, no doubt, at one time or another heard of the use of hypnotism in medical cases. If you haven't you must have been living in a cave or had your head in a barrel. For goodness sake, try at least to keep up with current events! Hypnotism has been used in many, many medical situations, such as in the cure of Phobias. John Phobia was cured of something by the use of hypnotism, as was his distant cousin, May Belle Phobia of Atlanta, Georgia. So, that makes it plan that Phobias are cured by the use of hypnotism.

Fat and Chance experimented in the uses of hypnotism for weight control. Fat would first attempt to hypnotize Chance, then vice-versa (or it may have been the other way around.) Usually, Fat's eyes would go into a glazed look, and just when Chance thought Fat was going under, Fat would get tickled and start chuckling. Then Chance would break into laughter, so they did not have too much success with hypnotism themselves. Nevertheless, this is being included, in event you try everything else and still find yourself to be fat. The way it works is this: Get someone to hypnotize you. This is usually done by the hynotizer swinging a railroad watch gently, to and fro, in front of your eyes, and repeating, "You are getting sleepy…sleepy."

If you do not have a railroad watch, you will have to try another diet.

Assuming you do have a railroad watch, have the party hypnotize you and tell you that when you wake up, you will eat very, very little. Be especially careful that you choose carefully the party to hypnotize you. (A word of warning!) Mrs. D.Q. of Hampton, New York (Case 458890) had her nephew Charlie, who is a practical joker such as you would not believe, hynotize her. The little devil told her, instead, that she would wake up very, very hungry. As soon as her eyes opened, she rushed to the refrigerator, downed a gallon of milk, half a bar-b-cued chicken, and a sack of brownies. Yes, a big joke for Charlie! So, be careful that the potential hynotizer is not a practical joker, or some kind of creep with romantic ideas.

One advantage to this diet is that, if one goes under very deeply, one may have some dental work or perhaps minor surgery done at this same time. (Let's face it, today a dollar is a dollar.)

Now, you say, what if you try this hypnotism idea, but it does not work for you? There are two other things we can do. One, you can have someone hypnotize you into thinking that you are thin. If you must remain fat, at least you will think you are thin. If you do this, however, it would be better if someone buys your clothes for you. You can see why.

The final alternative is to become very skilled in hypnosis yourself. Then, proceed to hypnotize everyone you meet into thinking that you are thin. Remember, if you choose this plan, to obtain a good railroad watch and to swing it in front of you wherever you go. Someone is bound to get hypnotized sooner or later!

THE AMAZING MUSHROOM DIET

Webster defines mushroom as "an enlarged complex aerial fleshy fruiting body of fungus." Uggghhh! That makes them sound terrible, doesn't it? Not only that, but that definition is an unbelievable difficult tongue-twister. (If you don't believe me, try to say it rapidly three times in succession.)

No matter. We all know what the mushroom is. Some like them, some do not. If you do like the little rascals, don't bother trying this diet. If you don't like them, you will probably eat very little and of course will lose weight. (Some people dislike them so much that they only pretend to eat them, and instead slip them beneath the tablecloth, and drop them to the floor.) If you do this, you will lose more weight.

One note of caution:

If you choose to pick your own mushrooms, be alert as some mushrooms will make you fatally ill. These are the deadly ones. Others are scrumptious and will leave you licking your fingers. We should now explain which are which. To be truthful, we have no idea how to tell one from the other.

Well, assuming you purchase some, or manage to pick the lucky ones, stay on the mushrooms only, and remain on the diet for thirty days. If you haven't lost any weight, stay on it for a year or two. After several years without success, forget it. This diet is obviously not going to do one bit of good. We will think of something else.

The diet has worked for many people, however. Let's look at a recent survey for the exact statistics.

16% of those trying the diet passed away, having picked the wrong mushrooms.

37% could never figure out how to prepare them.

46% ate the darn things for years, and exactly

50% of those gained weight, with the others neither gaining nor losing.

That makes 99%, so apparently we were wrong somewhere in our figures. Go back up to the sixteen-percent and make it read seventeen if it is all that important to you. Must you be so exactly perfect in everything? Picky, picky!

Well, if the diet works at all, it is because no one in their right mind would want to have mushrooms for breakfast, so they do not eat at all. Then, having had them for lunch, one certainly could not face them again for dinner!

Whatever your conclusions about mushrooms as a diet, when we began this book we felt we should include the mushroom diet. Now, we are not so sure. If you choose to, simply tear out these pages.

It was all a mistake anyway. What we were thinking of was a <u>muskmelon</u> diet. What could make one make such an error? There is scarcely any resemblance between the mushroom and the muskmelon. Or if there is, we fail to see it. What do you think?

THE AMAZING AIR DIET

It is now time to review. If you do not wish to review, you may run ahead to later chapters. Frankly, you will be missing something. Sometimes reviewing can be the best part. Are you still with us? Recall, then, that we have covered the Introduction to Fat and Chance, The Amazing Running Diet, The Amazing Blindfold Diet, The Amazing Hypnotism Diet, and finally thank goodness, The Amazing Mushroom Diet. Are you thinner yet? If not, we will go on until you are as thin as you wish to be, as you are in your wildest dreams. You will turn heads! (Perhaps you already do, but for the wrong reason!) We are talking about turning the heads of young men, who, when you have walked past, will whistle or perhaps say, "Va-va-voom," or something of that nature.

At this point, if you perhaps have not shed thirty or forty pounds, you may be getting discouraged, and saying things such as "This stupid Fat-Chance foolishness is hogwash!" Here, we suggest you call Raquel Welch or Brooke Shield. How do they look to you? When they answer the telephone (or your letter), they will of course claim they have never been on the Fat-Chance Diet. Would you expect them to admit it? Are you so foolish as to think they want the entire world to know the secrets of the stars? They do not want you going down the street looking like they do.

Millions of dollars have been spent by certain persons to keep this book from ever getting into print. If not millions, then surely thousands, or hundreds. Remember, too, that years from now, the book you hold in your hands will be extremely valuable, possibly priceless. Why? Because most will have been foolishly discarded, either before or after being read. And when there are only one or two left, you know that means.

Now, see what you have done. We have gotten off on some sort of tangent. This chapter is supposed to be on The Amazing Air Diet! The Air Diet is another of the plans in the Fat-Chance System, and was developed in the earlier days of Fat and Chance's collaboration. This would have been during the late forties. Then, you may recall, people thought it was rather nice to be plump. It showed, for one thing, that you had money or you could never have bought the kind of groceries it takes to be really chubby.

So, as Fat and Chance published their first diets, no one was at all interested. In fact, their first diet book sold only four copies. Fat and Chance and their mothers all bought one. So, times were hard. Fat and Chance themselves were penniless and had not a bite to eat in the small apartment they shared in the Bronx.

At last, one evening, Chance returned home from trying to get his mother to buy another diet book, only to find Fat sorely depressed and starved.

Said Fat, "Whatever shall we eat?"

Thinking aloud, which is not easy to do, Chance replied with more than a touch of sarcasm, "I suppose, my friend, that we shall eat <u>air</u>."

At that, Fat's eyes lit up, either from sheer hunger, or from the fact they had hit upon something. And they had hit upon, of course, The Amazing Air Diet.

In a seminar arranged at one of New York's finest stores, Fat and Chance illustrated that one may sit at the dinner table, and rather than heap one's plate, merely spoon out air, then munch as one normally would. After a few days of this, Fat and Chance found that the diet worked as well or better than <u>any</u> being touted. And it still does! One word of caution: it is better to practice this diet in private. One lady from Boston went to lunch with her club, and when she proceeded to spoon nothing but air into her plate, her friends quietly slipped behind her and tied her hands and took her for admission into the psychiatric ward at Community Hospital.

A letter from her recently indicated she is still there in the ward, but, mind you, she boasts of a sleek one hundred and two pounds, and wears a size five.

THE AMAZING TURKEY DIET

What would you think of a turkey diet? That is exactly what Fat and Chance thought when the idea was suggested to them! There are, of course, many critics of the turkey diet. One man from Oregon was heard to remark, "That takes the cake, doesn't it? Why in hell would any fool want to put turkeys on a diet? Turkeys are meant to be fat! Can you imagine Thanksgiving with the family gathered around the traditional table, and there in the midst would be a skinny turkey?"

Well, we must agree with him. Not that we must, really, because we can do darn well as we please. Let's say that we want to agree with him. At any rate, if one were to desire to put turkeys on diets, where would one begin? Probably a lettuce diet with lots of exercise, but then turkeys <u>never</u> exercise. They would look foolish if they did. And they will turn their heads away from lettuce with a look that says, "You have got to be kidding!"

Dr. Leonard Grossmann of New Jersey wrote us to suggest that what Fat and Chance had in mind is that <u>people</u> diet <u>on</u> turkey, rather than the turkeys themselves attempting to diet. Grossmann is a veterinarian and should keep out of it altogether. That is all we will say about the Amazing Turkey Diet. And none too soon we might add.

THE ONE MINUTE DIET

Since everything is instant these days, it seems that we should include the One Minute Diet in this book. Before we begin, though, let's set the record straight and clear up any misunderstandings. A Mrs. W. G. of Turtle Creek, Texas wrote in very excited about the diet. She thought she would only have to diet one minute a week! Isn't that the craziest thing you ever heard of? Obviously the lady had fallen on her noodle at some point to be that foggy!

Surely anyone would realize that with the One-Minute Diet one can only eat for one minute a week. (Two may eat for two minutes, of course, if you add their individual eating time together, but this is a diet book and not a math book, so we will not mention that again.)

This is one of those delightful diets where one may eat anything one desires, but the catch is that you must confine your weekly food intake to one minute. You each week have sixty seconds from the word "Go!" to gobble up anything that gets in your way.

Several rules must be followed. Failure to follow any single rule will result in your having to begin again at Day

One in the Fat – Chance Diet. Failure to follow two of the rules will result in suspension of your driver's license.

Rule #1:   You must eat with both hands tied behind your back. (Dieting is tough!)

Rule #2:   You may have no one assist you by plopping food into your mouth.

Rule #3:   If you eat for even one skinny second, one fraction of a moment longer than sixty seconds, your one minute will be reduced to only thirty seconds the next week. Further, a letter of reprimand will be sent to your parents, and a copy placed in your permanent file. So, don't be foolish! Watch the clock! It may be advisable to have a timekeeper, who will sound a gong to provide a five-second warning to that you can taper off and be certain not to over-run your time.

A Mr. R. W. of San Pedro, California (Case #181862) tried to get around Rule #2 by having another heavy dieter assist by placing sandwiches into his mouth, but the rascal ate the sandwiches himself, and a friendship was ruined for the sake of a few morsels. Another cheater, Mr. T.C.M. of

Pebble Beach (Case #7614-A) tried to cheat by having a neighbor help, and the neighbor was admitted to Pebble Beach Memorial Hospital with severe lacerations of the fingers.

One other word of caution: If you plan to align a row of goodies, be sure that nothing but food is in front of you! A terribly fat attorney from Tulsa, Oklahoma failed to remove some legal briefs from his dining table. He was dozing when a friend shouted "Go!" The obese attorney bolted to the table, consuming mass quantities of beef, at least a dozen ice cream sundaes, three boxes of chocolates, and unfortunately, all the briefs. His client ended up losing the case, and the last we heard had filed suit against the attorney for eating his defense. (Can you blame him?)

The one-minute diet can be tricky!

DAY ONE

We now come to the key program of them all, the Amazing 30-Day Fat-Chance Diet. We call this diet by the name we do because it is amazing, because it takes thirty days, and because Fat and Chance created the diet, with Fat doing the lyrics and Chance writing the musical score. (Notice the entire diet is in B Sharp Minor, and is scored for full orchestra including timpani.) Certain characters appearing in the diet are totally fictitious, and are not intended to represent any person either living, dead, or any other possible state.

The original copy of the diet was written on a paper napkin, as Fat and Chance dined at Mama Rosa's Restaurant in Rome, Italy. The diet was written at about 7:30 in the evening on April 22, 1978. (Chance had spaghetti with meat sauce, while Fat had fettucinni.)

The diet disappeared when Fat accidentally wiped his chin with the napkin containing the diet, and discarded it. It surfaced, miraculously, just this year when a Butcher in the Bronx (a guy named Vinny) spotted the napkin among the salami. Mere chance (no pun intended) saved the diet from being lost to society forever. Many speculate on how, in the name of heaven, the napkin managed to end up in the Bronx; others could not care less.

Now that you have been given some of the history of this remarkable diet, you have no more excuses! It is time to get down to the serious business of the diet itself. You have put it off and put it off, and now the time has come to take it off! This diet must be followed to the letter. It will be better if, during these thirty days, you talk to no one. Concentrate only on the diet. Do not go on dates, play the banjo, take night courses, or figure your income tax. Preferably, pull your shades, quit your job, wear dark sunglasses and a wig, and be doubly sure that you are not followed!

We start with Day One since it is the first day. If we were to start with Day Two we would already be one day and as much as five pounds behind (no pun intended.)

DAY ONE

Nothing

You read correctly. The first day eat nothing. If we start you off with a bunch of junk you will <u>never</u> start dieting. It is better to start right, to get off on the right foot, as they say. Whatever you do, do not stomp your foot and demand food, for if you do, according to the rules of the diet, you will have the same thing for Day Two.

DAY TWO

1 Grape

The grape, you will learn, plans an important role in the Fat-Chance Diet, and turns up from time to time. This is because of the following facts concerning the grape:

1. The grape is small. It only makes sense that eating a grape can do little harm to a diet.
2. The grape is generally easy to obtain, and is readily recognizable. The grape is usually round and is generally either green or purple, and approximately the size of a marble.

If you cannot recognize the grape, you are in trouble. Your problem is apparently optometric as well as dietary. What we mean is that you probably can't see the darn thing. Have your eyes checked promptly!

We said that the grape is easy to obtain. Sometimes that is not exactly true.

Take the case of Elvira M. of Gallup, New Mexico. Elvira, arriving at Day Two, had not a grape in the house. So, as one might expect, she got into her automobile (a Chevrolet, brown and white, with one hubcap missing on the right rear), and drove to the local supermarket, proceeding to the fruits and vegetables. Selecting a fine, plump grape, she carried it to the checkout.

"Madam," said the checkout (a rather smart-aleck fat little girl named Clarice), "You can't buy a single grape!"

Elvira was, as you might imagine, a bit irritated.

"And why in hell not?" she demanded.

The nasty little girl checkout replied that, for one thing, she has to weigh grapes, and the grape hardly registered on the scale, so you really didn't know what to charge. And certainly, she claimed, she couldn't just give Elvira the grape.

"Can you imagine what would happen if we just started giving away grapes?" shrieked Clarice.

Well, to make matters worse, Elvira demanded to see the store manager, and he turned out to be Clarice's father, and naturally took her side of the argument.

Finally, the Gallup police were called out, and Elvira was arrested for disorderly conduct. As soon as she is out of jail, she expects to resume her diet with Day Three.

DAY THREE

1   Macadamia Nut

2   Peas, Green

3   Drops of Coffee

And a Partridge in a Pear Tree

(We were only kidding about the partridge in the pear tree. Can't you take a joke? Besides the partridge is not allowed until the twenty-eighth day, or somewhere in there.) Not only that, but the chance of finding a partridge in a pear tree are a million to one. Partridges cannot stand pear trees, and will remain in one only if tied there. Even then, they set up such a racket you will live to regret ever putting them there in the first place.

The macadamia nut should be roasted for a day and a half, and the peas sautéed for not less than four hours. Much though has been given to making these meals tasty as well as nourishing, while taking the pounds off. So do not blow all of this by doing a sloppy job in the kitchen. Take some pride, for pete's sake! Sauté! Sauté!

If you wish, the coffee may be served one-third in the morning, one-third the afternoon, and the evening. If you choose to substitute tea for the coffee, you may do so, but the tea must be drunk at 2:12 p.m.

DAY FOUR

Well, how is it going? You have successfully completed three full days on the diet. Aren't you delighted? Aren't you thrilled to finally be on the way to a new thinner you? Aren't you <u>starved</u>?

Many people have this sensation, starving, at about this point in the diet. This is merely caused by the lack of food.

Here again, try to keep your mind off you-know-what. Now, admittedly, this is sometimes hard to do. Every time you turn around it seems you see a foot-long, a fantastic po-boy, or a banana split, heaped with fruit and topped with nuts and whipped cream. Above all, stay in control, stay at all times in absolute, total control. Never let your guard down for a moment. Alex K., in a classic case from our file, was just where you are, Day Four. Walking along 42nd Street in New York, Alex was trying to concentrate on anything but you-know-what. He was concentrating on taking little tiny steps, and counting them, as he walked up the street.

Then suddenly, without any warning whatsoever, a man rounded the corner eating a polish sausage on a bun.

Overcome by the aroma, Alex snatched the sausage from the man's hand, and stuffed it into his own mouth!

The man, incidentally, was dumbfounded and did nothing at all. Later, when interviewed, the man said that his first impulse had been to scream, but he realized people would have paid little attention to a man yelling, "Sausage! Sausage!"

You wish to know where your diet plan is for Day Four, don't you? Forgive us when we are getting carried away with these fascinating case histories.

3	Onions, Green
4	Ounces of Garlic
6	Sardines

Aren't you surprised? Aren't you amazed? This is the most food you have eaten in four days. Did you think we were going to let you starve completely? We are reasonable people.

You may notice that people may tend to avoid you after this meal. This is perfectly normal and is to be expected. In fact, this is purposefully done to keep people away from you. People, as you darn well know, continually try to get you to eat, eat, eat.

Aunt Minnie might say, "Oh, one piece of my German Chocolate Cake won't hurt you!"

Notice that Aunt Minnie is thin as a rail. She never eats the stuff herself. And I suppose she has no way of knowing that a true fatty can <u>never</u> eat "one piece" of anything!

Well, the menu for Day Four will certainly keep people away from you. There are some side effects which we will point out, as we usually do. One young man had his finance break their engagement after Day Four. Due to the rather strong odors, she could not enter his apartment at all. It was, however, not a totally sad case. The young man, on the same day, recognized the odor on a bus and met a young lady who, to their good fortune, was also on Day Four. They plan to be married on Day Twenty-Six and will serve that day's menu to their wedding guests. They had planned, as a romantic notion to serve the Day Four menu, but felt that perhaps the pastor and best man would feel the quarters were a bit close.

DAY FIVE

1   One-Quarter slice of bread (crust removed)

2   Tablespoons tea (Coffee may be substituted but must be frozen and eaten and must be saved for Day Six)

Did you think it was going to be easy? Did we ever say such a thing? No, from the beginning, you very well knew you were going to have to cut down to practically nothing. But look at the positive side, and see that here you are enjoying bread and tea. When you feel sorry for yourself, do two things. First, look in the mirror. Isn't that terrible! We should have left out the bread today, but we are just people, too, and feel like we should give you a break. The second thing to do is go back and look at the menu for Day One. If that doesn't make you feel better, nothing will! You will never have as bad a day as Day One. Almost as bad, but not exactly.

Here, we usually insert an anecdote, or case history, but we cannot think of one off-hand. Can you? Check back with us tomorrow (Day Six) and perhaps we can give you two case histories, making up for the one we missed today.

DAY SIX

1/16 Jalapeno Pepper

1 Teaspoon Bean Dip

Today's diet was suggested by Jose' Gonzalez of Tiajuana, Mexico. It is, essentially, a Spanish meal, of course, and is enhanced by a bit of Mexican music and perhaps antacid. This is the only, we repeat, only day of the diet when you may also have a small shot of tequila, and after lunch one may "siesta" until later in the afternoon.

As you see, as you near the end of our first week, we celebrate in the traditional Mexican style. Enjoy! But take care! It is at this point that many, many of you will falter, fall off the wagon. Yesterday we promised you case histories, and case histories you shall have.

Rosalie Juarez Garcia (not her real name), Case number 41699, reached Day Six doing quite nicely. Her brother Pedro (not his real name) helped her daily with her diet plan. If she asked for, say, on Day Four, more than the three green onions, her brother would say, "No, no." (He said this in Spanish, of course.)

Day Six posed a problem, however, when Rosalie turned to that page and saw the jalapeno pepper and bean dip. Rosalie swallowed the 1/16 pepper and teaspoon of bean dip, and her eyes suddenly glowed. She inquired (in Spanish, of course), "Beloved Brother, may I have more pepper and bean dip?" She fluttered her eyelashes and smiled sweetly.

"No, no" replied her brother Pedro, shaking his head and turning away as he always did.

It was a serious mistake, for Rosalie raised a large skillet high over her head, and bringing it down on Pedro's sombrero (which he was indeed wearing at the time). Pedro took an early siesta, and Rosalie promptly devoured thirty-two peppers, three large bowls of bean dip, forty-two tortillas, and a sopapilla.

It did not help her waistline, nor do any good to speak of for Pedro. So, learn something from this! If the sight of Mexican food drives you cuckoo, skip Day Six altogether.

We promised you two case histories today, but we are starving and must get something to eat. Perhaps tomorrow we will catch up on these case histories. They are really more of a pain than anything. But if you insist, we will try to dig up a few more.

DAY SEVEN

Well, can you believe it? You have now successfully completed the first full week of your diet. Call someone fatter than you and gloat a little. You might say something like this: "Madge, it's been a week now! I've lost (make up some number of pounds) and, would you believe, I really am not hungry!" Here, of course, you are lying, but perhaps the little white lie might help a real fatty to at least be encouraged enough to try. (Incidentally, Fat and Chance refer to these as little fat lies, rather than little white lies.)

Now, for Day Seven, you will actually, truly get to eat. You will not, of course, stuff yourself silly. We do not do that any more, do we? But we will eat three modest meals.

BREAKFAST

1/3 Apple

2 Tablespoons Sassafras Tea

LUNCH

1/8 Carrot, uncooked

DINNER

1 Filet Mignon

Did you notice something about breakfast and lunch? You didn't? Then go back and look again. Now, do you see it? Yes, you are right. This meal emphasizes fiber, or as some say, fibre. Say it.

Fiber is sometimes referred to as roughage. Sometimes not. Fiber is satisfying to one's hunger while being low in calories. Since it is so low in calories, go back if you wish and make that two carrots for lunch. Just take a pencil or pen and write in "2" where it says "1/8." Do not go changing numbers in this book harum-scarum! If we let you do that, you would change half the numbers in this book, or even more! Next thing we knew you would be changing carrot to carrot <u>cake</u>. Make only those changes that we instruct you to make! (You may, however, write your name in the front cover if you like.)

So, you notice that fiber is involved in the first two meals. Did you notice anything about the dinner meal? Go back right now and look. No, silly, it does not emphasize fiber! That was in breakfast and lunch. If you forget things that fast, how do you remember where you parked your car? No, the thing to notice about dinner is that it is a joke. You should have know that there is no way that you could have a filet mignon on Day Seven! The other diet writers would laugh us flat out of the business! Seriously, for dinner go back and repeat the third item of Day Four. Take our word for it that it is the best thing you could do now.

Forgive us for making a joke about the filet mignon. It was a dirty thing to do, and we will omit it from the next edition of the book. In fact, if you like, go back and mark through the mention of filet mignon. Go ahead, it's o.k. In fact, we feel so badly about making a joke about food to a hungry person, leave it in, and mark out the part about it being a joke. Just eat the damned thing, and get back with the diet tomorrow.

DAY EIGHT

Today will be a bit different. You may eat as much as you wish of today's food. Does that surprise you? Perhaps you are easily surprised. Anyway, here is today's food:

1 Rabbit

If you somehow have managed to not lose weight up to now, your day has come. Several features of today's diet plan guarantees a weight loss. First, you must catch a rabbit. If you think that is easy, you are in for a surprise indeed. For one thing, you must start out early in the morning and drive to a place where rabbits are likely to live, or at least, perhaps, be passing through. These would likely be areas where bushes, briar, weeds, brush—you get the picture.

Wear something comfortable, and preferably sneakers or track shoes.

If you live far from the woods or fields, you must not eat on either the day traveling to or the day traveling from the fields. (If you spend a day traveling, obviously Day

Eight will become Day Nine, and you will finish the Fat Chance Diet a day later. You figure it out and let us know.)

Some people have lost 30, 40, or even 50 pounds on Day Eight alone. In Case History #53239 a 440-pound man left Los Angeles on Day Eight which happened to fall on June 4. The man turned up near Las Vegas, Nevada on August 21, running past the Golden Nugget shouting to passersby, "Have you seen a little brown rabbit go by here?" He was down to ninety-seven pounds! The diet works.

There is a second way in which the diet may work if you are a lady. Many ladies, having spent a day or a week chasing rabbits, finally end up with, say, a cute little rabbit that they can't bear to cook, and instead give it to grandchildren for Easter. So, not only have they gotten some exercise, but also managed to pass up Day Eight eating nothing at all.

DAY NINE

1/50 Ounce Bamboo Shoots

1/3 Shrimp (small)

2 Ounces Tea

Aren't you pleased? A Chinese dinner! You probably thought when you started this diet that you would hardly be enjoying your favorite foods. To further the festive atmosphere you might want to invite a Chinese person over. Be certain, however, that this is a fat, dieting Chinese individual, or you might offend him. First, he might be offended by such meager quantities. (It will be permissible to double the menu portions if you have a guest, provided you do not try to eat both portions yourself. This is an old, old chubby person's trick. Usually, they will say to the guest, "You probably don't want any of this, do you?")

The second way in which one might offend a Chinese guest is that perhaps he is not dieting and would bring along immense bowls of sweet and sour pork and vast containers of rice and vegetables. Then, if you do not eat, surely he will be puzzled and quite possibly offended. You are, of course, caught between a rock and a hard place, so to speak. If you eat all that stuff, you will balloon back up, and we must remind you, have to start all over again at Day One. Perhaps it will be better not to invite anyone after all.

DAY TEN

This is one of those days in which you may have as much of the menu item as you wish. No kidding. While it would be preferable to eat only perhaps a half cup, you may indeed eat all you wish. The dish for today is carrot ice cream.

"What," wrote one lady from New Orleans, Louisiana, "is carrot ice cream?"

Another lady, this one from Miami, Florida, and apparently a lady with extreme poor vision, wrote us, "What is parrot ice cream?" (Apparently she misread the "c" as a "p.") She may have something there! While we have never heard of parrot ice cream, that does not necessarily mean that there is no such thing. (There are lots of things we haven't heard of...how about you?)

Well, to answer the first question, carrot ice cream is merely strawberry ice cream, made with carrots in the place of strawberries. (If we had intended to have you eat strawberry ice cream, we would have said so. No, we are talking about carrot ice cream here.)

Again, there are certain precautions. When we say that you may eat all you want, try to be half-sensible about it! J. R. T. of Mesquite, Texas started on the Fat-Chance Diet, got to Day Ten, and went completely bananas! The man made twenty gallons of carrot ice cream, and ate the entire thing! Not only did he balloon up in weight, but his stomach turned orange. We had to send him straight back to Day Four, with a warning that another occurrence of this nature would result in his having to skip Day Ten altogether and have no carrot ice cream at all.

Here is a tip: Many dieters enlist a friend to assist them. It works like this: Have a friend monitor your progress. If necessary instruct the friend to give you the day's meal, and only that not one bite more. Tell them that, if you insist on more than the allowance, to ignore you. Tell them to pretend that they do not hear you. Suggest they play a cello or something loudly with their back to you. Tell them that, under no circumstances, no matter how you yell or stomp your feet, are they to allow you one whit more. Tell them not to be surprised if you call them a rather nasty name, or kick their shins, or attempt to throttle them with their own necktie. (One word, now to the friend who is helping: The only time that you must concede the point and allow the dieter to have more than the daily allowance is in the case where the dieter produces a pistol. Now, often this is done in bluff, and the weapon is merely a child's toy, or at worst is unloaded. But there are limits to which a dieter's friend is expected to go. Hence, when a dieter does produce a weapon, it is perhaps better to say something such as, "Ha, ha, Fred, I was only <u>joking</u>. I really had you going there for a while, didn't I? Have some ice cream!" This is all covered, incidentally, in our companion book, <u>What To Do When Your Best Friend Diets</u>.)

DAY ELEVEN

Today one may have a truly royal diet. Then again, one may not. It all depends. Though Fat and Chance developed this menu, it is, in essence, the same menu enjoyed by His Highness, King Louis the XV of France, according to all available records of the royal diet, or at least what we have heard.

Louis the XV (or it could have been another Louis altogether, as the records are very sketchy) tended to overeat. On one occasion, he was overhead to say, "Nowaways the King will have a snack.." (Here historians differ. Historians differ a lot. More than they should, in our opinion. At any rate, some scholars feel that the King used the word "nowadays" and not "nowaways" which sounds rather silly. Other scholars feel that he did say "nowaways," but that he said "steak" not "snack," which is a fairly modern word, and he would never have thought of it.) Where are we in this story, and how did we get into it anyway? Oh yes, Louis was overheard to say that he was going to eat a small meal. He then proceeded to eat three baked game hens, five loaves of fresh-made bread, a large jar of olives, and, accidentally of course, there proclamations he was to have read later in the day. Like so many heavy folk, the King had no awareness of his bulk. Upon entering the throne room after the massive meal, the King plopped himself onto the throne, whereupon the left two legs gave away, the throne tilting sharply to the left, tumbling the King onto the floor. The King was uprighted by means of a clever device improvised by the King's engineers. They termed it a "Louis Lever" and such devices may be referred to even today in such a way. However, they may not be. Please remember that this is a diet book and not an engineering book! How do you expect us to know <u>everything</u>?

Well, anyway, on the following day the King immediately determined to lose the massive girth he was known for, and he began a special diet. At this point we would like to present that diet. We would like to but we cannot, for two reasons, really. The first reason is that we have taken so long with this story that we are going to have to move on to Day Twelve or we will never get through this diet.

The second reason is that we can't make it out. Whatever the King ate is scribbled out on a sort of parchment and is smudged by what appears to be blueberry jam. The word describing the King's primary food appears to be either a four letter word beginning with the letter "q" or a seventeen letter word ending in "z.." See what you can make of it.

DAY TWELVE

BREAKFAST
1 Raspberry

LUNCH
1 Cup Lobster Thermidor

DINNER
2 Grapes (Medium-size)

Doubtless you were surprised to see lobster thermidor on your menu. You should not be surprised, for lobster is nutritious, a good protein food, and is impressive to your neighbors. ("I'll have the lobster," sounds good in restaurants. Try it.) But expensive! Sakes alive! Small wonder you can have only one cup! If it suits you financially, take your pencil and mark out the lobster and write in tuna fish. Careful not to mark out the raspberry, by mistake, or you will be stuck with seafood for breakfast and lunch.

We must request, also, that you do not request to substitute wine for the fruit selection for dinner. At one time we allowed this on day Twelve, but had to discontinue that. One gentleman (J.K. of St. Louis, Missouri, as I recall) made that request in writing, and we verified that it would be permissible. What did he do? He skipped all the way from Day One to Day Twelve, marked out "2 Grapes" and penciled in "2 Quarts Rose," then repeated Day Twelve seventeen times. Then and there we decided there would be no substitutions on Day Twelve other than the tuna fish, and we also made the firm rule we reminded you of earlier about penciling things into your diet. Doodle if you must, but never change the menu unless we specifically tell you to do so. If you must doodle, be careful that you do not absentmindedly doodle ice cream cones or hamburgers or that kind of thing. If you need a list of things to doodle that make no reference to food, write us. We will not send you a list, but writing us may help take your mind off food.

DAY FOURTEEN

You say that you noticed there was no diet plan for Day Thirteen? Certainly not! Surely you know that buildings have no thirteenth floor, and you should very well know why. Thirteen is the unlucky number. We, in fact, intended to omit the number thirteen from appearing anywhere in this book. Go back and check. (If we did somehow let one sneak in, please take your pencil and mark it out.)

In our studies, many, many people have reported most unusual and unfortunate things happening to them when they had a Day Thirteen in their diet plan. Take the case of Mrs. T. M. of Goose Bay, Ontario. Mrs. T.M. was permitted, in that particular diet, on that particular day, to have a grape. (It was a green seedless.) Well, the grape slipped from her fingers, rolled across the floor, under the door and onto the front porch. We should note that Mrs. T.M. was wearing only the briefest of underthings, and normally would not have even considered going out dressed in that fashion. But it <u>was</u> the thirteenth day, and she was hungry to say the least. Opening the door a small crack, she could see the grape resting only a couple of feet outside the door. Overcome by hunger, Mrs. T.M. threw open the door and dashed onto the porch. As she felt her foot slip on the grape, she also heard the door slam shut behind her.

We could end the story right there, but since you paid good money for this book, we will go ahead and tell you the rest of it.

With considerable discomfort in the area of her lower back, Mrs. T.M. got up, and realizing the locked status of the door, and her attire, or lack of it, raced to the window and was attempting to pry it open when a prowl car happened by. When she attempted to explain the whole thing, the grape having rolled under the door, etc., she was hauled in.

"Thirty dollars or thirty days!" roared the judge, who himself was dieting and in a lousy mood. Dressed as she was, Mrs. T.M. had no money on her, and very little else.

We could tell you some stories! But you get the idea why Day Thirteen was skipped altogether.

DAY FIFTEEN

Oh, no! We seem to have done it again! Did you notice that we gave you no diet plan on Day Fourteen? That would not be so bad except for the fact that there was no Day Thirteen. (You must be pretty hungry.) We will prescribe a diet today that will delight you...well, perhaps not delight you, but it couldn't be worse than Day Fourteen, could it?

Forgetting to include something to eat on Day Fourteen reminds us of a funny story, or perhaps we shouldn't say "funny." Let's just say a story. These stories appear to be very important to dieters. While they appear to be, they are not, however. If you want to skip this story, drop on down to the diet for the day. But do not skip any other portion of this book, unless we specifically tell you to. And we do not do that very often. Now and again we may. Where were we?

Oh, yes, in a diet book released in 1978, the printer inadvertently left out fifteen pages, and the poor dieters skipped from Day Ten to Day Twenty-five. How mad they are were! But thin, at least! Checking into this incident, we found that the printer was a huge dude named Frank from Columbus, Ohio, who did not believe in dieting. In fact, he hated dieting. And it showed! One entire section of the book was printed upside down, and the readers had to stand on their heads to even read it. Already weak from hunger, many dieters did not have the strength to right themselves again, and a few are reported, even now, to still be standing upside down.

And that was not the worst of it! Many people, after paying nearly ten bucks for the book found gravy stains throughout and could hardly make out the diet at all. One lady, a Mrs. Q.M. from Uvalde, Texas, encountered a particularly stained page and, rather than the word "salad," made a word out to be "salaf," which, strangely enough is an actual word from a now lost ancient Arabic tongue, a word which means "great feast." Luck would have it that, of all dieters, this woman knew a smattering of the dialect. As puzzled as she was, she followed instructions (as good dieters always do.) She began setting forth for herself a great meal. Heaping bowls of pork, immense platters of pasta, and elegant trays of fine pastries. She gained thirty-six pounds over the next few days. Do not think that printers are not important. Try to purchase diet books, if you can, printed by dieting printers, because they will take far greater care. Also check for gravy stains on the pages.

You probably thought we had again forgotten to give you your daily diet plan, but no indeed!

BREAKFAST

| 1 Teaspoon | Scrambled Egg |
| 1/3 | Fried Banana |

LUNCH

| 2 Bowls | Raw Squid |

DINNER

1	Sparerib, Pork
1 Piece	Peanut Brittle
1 Tablespoon	Cottage Cheese

Notice that you are actually eating! In the event you have forgotten how: one places the food into one's mouth, then chews, and swallows. Some diets are so bad people forget how to eat. It is important that we explain why these particular items were selected for Day Fifteen. First, you should note that you are now half-way through the Thirty Day Plan of the Fat-Chance Diet. Congratulations! By now you should have lost considerable pounds. If you haven't, go back to Day One and start all over. You must have been cheating on the diet. How could you do such a thing? Shame on you!

If you have lost the weight, you deserve a lot of credit. You will find that you feel better and that your sex life has improved. You don't and it hasn't? Well, for goodness sake, don't expect everything! Maybe at least you can get into some clothes you wore last year before you let yourself get all out of shape.

Where were we? Oh yes, we were saying that it is important that you understand how these particular items were selected for Day Fifteen. Mainly, scrambled eggs were selected because there aren't too many things people have for breakfast, so it was that or cereal, and we needed cereal for Day Sixteen. The rest of the stuff was stuff that people do not like, usually. At least, that is the case for the fried banana and (ugh!) the raw squid. People, we find, will pass up items if they are pretty bad. (We will be using some others that are really bad later on.)

Now, as to the pork sparerib, we meant to tell you to scrape away <u>all </u>meat, leaving only the bone, which may be chewed on. (Surely you did not think we would be foolish enough to put a pork sparerib on a diet!)

The peanut brittle was added on the diet because it tends to get between the teeth and be such a bother that people will tend to pass it by, too. (The idea, as we say, is that the more you pass up, the thinner you get.) That is not a problem, because at some point people get so hungry they will eat <u>anything</u>, so they surely will not starve even on a lousy diet.

Well, let's wrap up Day Fifteen. The cottage cheese was placed on the menu because all diets <u>must</u> contain cottage cheese, although no one seems to know why. Apparently it is a federal law of some kind, like kidnapping and interstate transporting of stolen goods. So there it is. Some diets, incidentally, go completely wild on cottage cheese. We suspect these diet books are published by people who also own cottage cheese companies. Either that or college boys playing pranks. At any rate, from time to time, so as not to alienate anyone, we will put some cottage cheese on the diet. You do not have to eat it.

DAY SIXTEEN

This is going to be a most unusual day! Not because of the diet, but because of your horoscope. All of the signs look fairly strange for this particular day. Many people are surprised to find us making mention of their horoscope. Frankly, so are we. But we feel that we do not only have an obligation to assist you in your diet, but also to help you to become better educated, more polished, a better scrabble player, and a good loser, among other things. That is a lot to get out of a cheap book. Nowadays the price of this book will buy you nothing.

Today, we have to use cereal for breakfast since eggs were used yesterday, and pancakes and syrup are out of the question.

BREAKFAST

1 Serving   Cereal

LUNCH

2 Tablespoons   Cottage Cheese

DINNER

The meat from that sparerib from yesterday, if you have not thrown it away or given it to the dog. (We thought it over and felt it was cruel to make a person scrape a sparerib and gnaw on the bone. It was never our intention to be cruel—diets just seem to come out that way.)

DAY SEVENTEEN

At this point in the diet, in all fairness to you, we must explain that a portion of the original Fat-Chance Diet was lost. That was Day Seventeen and the better portion of Day Eighteen. Well, the pages were not actually lost. They were in fact eaten by an irate typist named Elvira who worked for Fat and Chance. After months of disgust over what Fat and Chance were paying her, and as she prepared those pages, Elvira lost her temper, kicked over the typewriter, tore Days Seventeen and Eighteen into shreds and popped them into her mouth. (She also had the nerve to stuff Day Nineteen into Fat's mouth and Day Twenty into Chance's mouth, while chanting "You cheap so-and-so's!" These pages were retrieved, and you will find Nineteen and Twenty as they were originally prepared.)

As for Day Seventeen, we can't think of anything offhand. If you can stand it, have some cottage cheese. Otherwise just see what is in the refrigerator, but DO NOT OVERDO IT!

If you can't be trusted to go into the refrigerator by this time, and not make a pig of yourself, we do not have, apparently, a very good relationship established. If you are afraid to go to the refrigerator by yourself, have one of your parents or a good friend go with you.

DAY EIGHTEEN

As you may recall from Day Seventeen, the original diet plan for that day and for Day Eighteen was lost to us. If you do not recall that, you have a memory problem that is far greater than your weight problem, and you should be spending your time and money on that problem. We may take up the problem of memory later in this book, but it doesn't seem likely. Then, again, if we remember to, we might. Don't be surprised either way.

BREAKFAST
1 Cup   Gooseberries

LUNCH
1 Chicken Gizzard

DINNER

*If you last name is Schmidt or Hauftenzeller or something like that, you may substitute 1/3 cup of sauerkraut or, if this day falls mid-week, perhaps a half a frankfurter. On the other hand, if your name is Gonzales or similar, and you choose, you may have a second tortilla instead of the chicken gizzard. If you are of Cajun heritage (you will know this by your name, which we be something like Arceneaux or Boudreaux), you may have a tiny cup of crab gumbo both for lunch and dinner. Please, no other substitutions, and remember that <u>everyone</u> must eat the gooseberries.

DAY NINETEEN

BREAKFAST
1 Wedge   Melon

LUNCH
1 Slice   Beef Tongue

DINNER
1 Tablespoon   Passionfruit

Many people have written us about one wedge of melon. That shows that people have too much time on their hands if they have nothing better to do than write letters about wedges of melon. But, to get on with it, the most frequently asked question is, "What do I do with the rest of the melon?" That is a good question.

Other letters we receive are concerning the beef tongue. (Our letters are rather boring, if you haven't realized that already.) "Why do you offer the beef tongue?" people ask. Who do you know that likes beef tongue? We must remind you that diets must largely be made up of stuff that people hate, or they would eat so much it would be worse than being on no diet at all.

We threw in the passionfruit because of the sound of it. We have no idea what it is, but it has a great name. Say it three times rapidly and you will see what we mean. Besides, a tablespoon of <u>anything</u> couldn't put much weight on you.

DAY TWENTY

BREAKFAST

¼   Raisin

LUNCH

1 Slice   Ham

DINNER

The Other ¾

of the raisin.

It is important to properly prepare the meals above. Well, if not important, let's say it wouldn't be a bad idea.

As to the raisin, it should be baked at 336° for approximately six hours. If it comes out absolutely black and hard as a rock, 336° may be a little high, so start over. If you plan to eat at precisely noon, then you'd obviously have to have the raisin in the oven by six a.m. If you plan to eat earlier, say at eleven a.m., then you must begin cooking at five, which seems pretty ridiculous! But then, that is your business.

Come dinner, many dieters complain they cannot find the rest of the raisin. (Writing a diet book is not easy! You have to put up with all kinds of thing!) One lady, returning to where she thought she had left the raisin, instead swallowed a small black bug that had crawled onto the countertop, while another (Mrs. H.B. of Shinrock, Arizona, Case #37940) swallowed a button. At least she thinks it was a button.

How about that big, thick and juicy slice of ham? Do you think we would let you get away with that? Hunger must have made you delirious! This ham slice must be thin. We are talking <u>thin</u>! When you think you have a thin slice, cut it in two again, and twice more. You must be above to see completely through this piece of ham! It must be completely transparent! Now, probably what will happen is that you will get frustrated trying to slice the ham. Don't be too hard on yourself, for you are only human. We all do the same on Day Twenty. Expect to get aggravated. Plan to be annoyed. In eighty-six percent of the cases studied, the dieter cut someone else close by. Perhaps the most extraordinary statistic is that in <u>every</u> case—<u>every</u> case, mind you—the ham was thrown on the floor, and, in sixty-eight percent of the cases, stomped on with the feet. In almost all the cases (where it could be found) the raisin portion remaining was also thrown to the floor.

You can see, the dieter is usually too frustrated at this point to eat at all, and most will not eat for several days. You will lose weight on the diet, as well as possibly a finger.

DAY TWENTY-ONE

BREAKFAST

1/59   Papaya

LUNCH

1/43   Guava*

DINNER

1/68   Pineapple

Notice how festive you feel on Day Twenty-One, and, of course, how hungry! But you will feel festive today because of the special tropical fruit menu. Close your eyes as you dine and you will envision yourself on a tropical beach with palm trees, crystal clear waters, and ukulele music wafting on the breeze. You will be doing great until you try to cut 1/59 of a papaya! Today will actually be worse than Day Twenty. (Remember the transparent ham?) If you don't remember the transparent ham, it may be because you are cheating on this diet! If you are skipping days, woe be unto you when we catch you! If you think you can jump through the diet four and five days at a time, you are loco. You won't lose weight, silly. Now, if you have cheated, go back and make up those days. We will sit right here and wait for you. Gad!

DAY TWENTY-TWO

BREAKFAST

1/8 Teaspoon   Grapejuice

LUNCH

1 Teaspoon   Butterbean Shavings

(in sauce)

DINNER

Apple Peel

You probably notice today is kind of tough. Well, it has to be! Don't you see what day it is? Only eight more days! How time flies!

To instruct you as to preparation of today's meals:

The juice should first be extracted from the grape. More often than not, this is done by means of a small incision on the right side of the grape. (Please do not write in asking which is the right side. If the grape appears to be backward, merely grasp the grape between the thumb and forefinger, and turn the grape around.) Use the same thumb-and-forefinger approach to gently squeeze the juice from the grape.

A second technique is to elevate the grape above one's head and squeeze the juice directly into your mouth. Our advice, based on experience, is: don't. In seventy-two percent of the tests conducted, the juice went into the eye rather than the mouth.

Do not—repeat, do not—eat the grape! Has anyone instructed you to eat the grape? If not, then why have you eaten it? If you have eaten the grape, you've just eaten tomorrow's breakfast! (The grape should be returned to the refrigerator for use on Day Twenty-three.) Incidentally, you may wish to apply a small piece of tape over the incision on the grape's right side. This is to preserve whatever moisture is left in the grape. Nothing is worse than a <u>dry</u> grape! (Do not forget to remove the tape tomorrow.)

On to lunch! Shave the butterbean, and cook the shavings in one tablespoon of water for a few hours. Water may be added as you cook. (You may have some trouble finding a saucepan only an inch wide—but that is your problem.) The core of the bean? You guessed it! How smart you are! Fat, but smart! The core will be lunch tomorrow. Notice how we make use of all this food, so that none is wasted. This is a trick we learned from the American Indian. The American Indian we learned it from was Henry Walkslow of Tulsa, Oklahoma. We learned other tricks, of course, from the American Indian. We learned things such as how to sneak up behind a white man and knock him senseless with a tomahawk. But this is not done so much anymore. But then that is another subject altogether. Do you think we can cover American history and everything under the sun in one cheap little book? Good grief!

Wrap the core of the bean in a small piece of paper, and set it aside until tomorrow. It may be wise to attach a three-by-five card onto the wrapper, saying "bean" or something like that. Otherwise you may lose the tiny wrapped little package. It has been known to happen. And an angry dieter may assault a family member who has thrown away tomorrow's lunch. Next to marital infidelity, this is the most common cause of family disharmony.

DAY TWENTY-THREE

BREAKFAST

Grape (See yesterday.)

LUNCH

1 Teaspoon   Polar Bear Fat

DINNER

1 Glass   Bicarbonate in water

Remember to make use of that grape left over from yesterday's menu. There is no sense in wasting food. (If you got up during the night and ate the grape, go back to Day Twenty-One and come forward again. There can be no cheating on this diet, as you well know by now.)

Did you notice that lunch called for polar bear fat? This was thrown in because Eskimos are frequently over looked when diets are drawn up. And believe me, there are plenty of fat Eskimos who need to diet as much as you do! The bicarbonate is scheduled for dinner because many people don't care at all for polar bear fat, and have trouble with it.

We should add that procuring polar bear fat is not easy, and the experience you get in trying will surely take some weight off you. Polar bears are ill-tempered. Occasionally you can make a pet of one, if you want to take the chance.

DAY TWENTY-FOUR

1 Rabbit

Today's diet may seem familiar with you. It should. It is the same as Day Seven. We repeated this day's diet for several reasons. First, many people have asked that the day be repeated. At least one or two have, anyway. It was a good day, so let's do it again. (At this time turn back and reread your instructions for Day Seven.)

The second reason we are repeating Day Seven is that we are running out of ideas. If you have any ideas for the diet, you may send them to us. We will not read them, but you certainly may send them. It is still a free country.

If for some reason you do not wish to repeat Day Seven, you may repeat Days Three and Four, or any combination that adds up to seven. How much more liberal can you be? We are giving you a lot of slack in this diet.

DAY TWENTY-FIVE

BREAKFAST

1 Selection   Cereal Group

LUNCH

1 Selection   Vegetable Group

DINNER

1 Selection   Meat Group

Here we begin to give you some control over your diet. Here you begin selecting your foods from the basic groups. Study these groups and the foods that make them up. Authorities tell you that there are five basic food groups. They tell you lots of things, as well. And you probably pay them little mind.

Not only should you have five basic food groups in mind, but it would not hurt you to learn of various other groups such as Count Basie's band, and the Lions Club, just to name a couple.

DAY TWENTY-SIX

BREAKFAST

1 Selection   Milk Group

DINNER

1 Selection   Fruit Group

Notice that we continue today with the food groups. Are you still reading and learning of the food groups? Or wasting your time on TV soap operas and those tabloids you get from the grocery check-out counter? For goodness sake get going with this food group thing!

Notice, too, that we omitted lunch. If you were busy studying your food groups, as you should have been, you wouldn't have noticed that you missed lunch.

Since we are on the milk group, it is very interesting to note—well, not <u>very</u> interesting, but maybe a little interesting—that there were 22,935,000 milk cows on farms in the U. S. in the year 1948. There originally had been 22,935,001 milk cows on farms, but one cow was reportedly living within the city limits of Philadelphia at the time, and had to be omitted from the official count. Another fact, less interesting than the first, is that, on the night of October 17, 1948, at precisely 7:38 p.m., all the cows apparently mooed at the same moment, creating a rather terrible "moooo" all across the nation. The phenomena has not occurred again since that night! The cows apparently got a kick out of doing it once, but never bothered again.

DAY TWENTY-SEVEN

BREAKFAST
1/16   Pancake

LUNCH
3 Eyedroppers   Syrup

DINNER
Peanut

A word of caution here:

The peanut is a dangerous item to include in a diet, such as this one. It is similar, in many ways, to popcorn. Not that you would mistake one for the other, of course. (Popcorn is white and fluffy-looking; peanuts are brown, like small pellets within a soft shell. Do we have to tell you everything?)

But the similarity is that, once one commences eating peanuts or popcorn, one can hardly stop! And that makes it bad for one on a diet. Take Case No. 442-9, a certain Homer L. of Brooklyn, N.Y. Homer had done quiet well on his diet, and did indeed make it all the way to Day Twenty-Seven. To celebrate, he took his youngest son Leon to a game between the Yankees and the Dodgers. During the course of the game, Leon purchased a small bag of peanuts.

"Leon," the father inquired, "Might I have a peanut?"

"Certainly, Father," replied Leon, handing his father the bag. Upon eating a peanut, Homer's eyes sort of glazed over and he promptly popped a second, then a third into his mouth. Finally, the rest of the bag! By this time little Leon was crying and stamping his feet, trying to get the bag back. Homer, by this time, was totally out of control, and leaped over the crowd, tackling a vendor, and stuffing his pockets with the bags of peanuts. Reports were that, at final count, he had eaten twenty-nine bags. Watch out for the peanuts.

DAY TWENTY-EIGHT

Pear

On this day, while we have only one meal (from the fruit group), you may digest the entire pear. You need not eat the core unless you choose. But if you do, mark it down somewhere. You should always mark everything down somewhere. That would include old high school chums' phone numbers, grocery lists, etc.

In keeping with our practice in this book (and we do try to keep in practice), we will tell you something of the pear. Not only will you be thinner when you complete the book but you might know something as well. It can't hurt.

The importance of the pear (among tree fruits) is exceeded only the the apple. Many people who love pears resent that. But we are not getting into the controversy. We are just trying to tell you some facts. Do not blame us. To go on, Early Greeks ate pears. Late Greeks found there were no pears to be eaten, as the early Greeks had of course eaten them. France ordinarily leads all countries in pear production. Germany ranks second. This has caused some hard feeling over the years, and in 1927 resulted in a serious fight, with Germany finally surrendering, and both sides agreeing to help pick up the terrible mess of pears that had been thrown.

DAY TWENTY-NINE

Eat nothing at all today! We are heading down the final stretch. We want to wrap this diet up in good style. If you are absolutely dying for food, you may inhale vapors from the pots if someone is cooking in the house. It might be wise to have someone restrain you as you inhale, because vapor inhalation is often the undoing of the dieter. If you feel that you may be inclined to assault those restraining you, perhaps you will want to try a pair of Dieter Cuffs. These are simply some old used police handcuffs we have purchased and reconditioned. They may be applied with one end around an arm or ankle and the other around a table leg.

Don't give up now. If you blow it today, you will have to go all the way back to Day One!

DAY THIRTY

Well, they said you couldn't do it, didn't they? They scoffed and pointed fingers at you. But here you are. Aren't you thin? See how fat they are!

To celebrate the successful conclusion of the Fat-Chance Diet, we are going to let you fill in your own menu yourself today! Congratulations!

BREAKFAST

....
....
....
....
....

LUNCH

....
....
....
....
....

DINNER

....

....

....

....

....

Dr. Hans Spud

Phyllis Diller

What do you expect of a diet book written by a guy named "Spud"? Dr. Potato has come up with a wonderful diet that I could stay on. The man is obviously bonkers with quite a breeze in the attic. But he IS thin and that is the whole idea. I have only slept with him twice and each time I lost 12 pounds. I recommend this diet to anyone over 93 or anyone living East of the Mississippi. Start the diet in January when Mars is straining steadily toward a vanilla Cusp. Depilatory rubbed on rye bread and thrown over the left shoulder hastens weight loss. So does drinking and dancing all night.

PHILLIS DILLER

ABOUT THE AUTHOR

Dr. Hans Spud, a native of Vienna, Austria, is founder of The Spud Institute. Dr. Spud is the author of the hilarious book *THE FAT-CHANCE DIET*, which has drawn raves from The Beaumont Enterprise, PM Magazine, and comedienne Phyllis Diller. As founder and director of the Spud Institute, the doctor makes news wherever he goes. The latest findings of the Spud Institute are made available to the news media in special press conferences and through the *Journal of the Spud Institute*.